I0697416

# Managing Osteoarthritis *during* Pregnancy

# Managing Osteoarthritis *during* Pregnancy

## Tips and Insights

Victoria Smith

# Dedication

In sincere tribute, this book is dedicated: to God for His grace and wisdom, my beloved family, the wonderful readers who'll discover connection in these pages, and to every incredible supporter who illuminated my path. Your steadfast faith has brought me to this point. A heartfelt dedication is reserved for all readers, especially those expectant mothers facing the challenge of osteoarthritis, pursuing well-being and recovery. Your journey holds significance, and this book stands as your companion.

# Table of Contents

# Acknowledgement

I want to express my heartfelt thanks to God for guiding me throughout the creation of this book. My family's unwavering support and the invaluable contributions of my editor, publisher, and collaborators have shaped its success. To my friends, your constant encouragement has meant the world.

For the amazing picture, a special thanks to timesofindia.indiatimes.com. Furthermore, I want to thank everyone who has read my work and appreciates it very much. I'm glad I got to experience it with you because it's been an amazing ride.

# Introduction

Pregnancy is a magnificent trip that is filled with expectation, joy, and a little bit of worry. It is a remarkable journey that brings new life to the world.

Imagine embarking on this beautiful voyage while also navigating the intricate pathways of osteoarthritis. This book, "Managing Osteoarthritis during Pregnancy: Tips and Insights," aims to provide you with a comprehensive guide on how to navigate the delicate balance between managing osteoarthritis symptoms and ensuring a healthy pregnancy. Drawing upon expert advice, medical insights, and practical tips, this resource is designed to empower you with the knowledge and tools needed to embark on this unique chapter of your life.

Pregnancy, with its miraculous transformations, can sometimes cast a shadow on the lives of those who battle osteoarthritis. Yet within these pages, you will discover a symphony of wisdom that harmonizes the rhythms of life-bearing love with the symphony of self-care. As you read on, you'll be immersed in a world where medical expertise meets compassionate understanding, offering you a comprehensive roadmap for embracing the journey ahead.

With insights gleaned from seasoned experts and real-life experiences, this book is more than just a guide; it's a reassuring companion on your path. You'll uncover invaluable tips, practical strategies, and a tapestry of stories that illuminate the way forward. From nutrition that nourishes both body and soul to exercises that honor your joints and nurture your spirit, each page unveils layers of guidance designed to empower you.

Let this book serve as the guiding light that clears away doubts, offers encouragement, and guides you into a world where your goals for joint health and parenthood are harmoniously intertwined. "Managing Osteoarthritis during Pregnancy: Tips and Insights" is more than simply a promise of solace; it's a call to embrace the extraordinary with grace, fortitude, and an uncompromising devotion to your wellbeing and that of your developing wonder.

# Chapter 1

# Understanding Osteoarthritis and Pregnancy

"Understanding Osteoarthritis and Pregnancy" is all about the connection between two important aspects: osteoarthritis and the experience of being pregnant. Osteoarthritis is a condition that affects the joints in our body, causing pain and stiffness. It often gets worse as we age, and it can make moving around more difficult. While Pregnancy, on the other hand, is a special time when a woman's body goes through many changes to support the growth of a new life inside her.

This chapter helps us make sense of how these two things relate to each other. It talks about how being pregnant can affect osteoarthritis and vice versa. For instance, the changes in hormones and the extra weight during pregnancy might make the symptoms of osteoarthritis better or worse.

Ultimately, the goal of understanding this connection is to make sure that people who are going through pregnancy and dealing with osteoarthritis have the right information and support. This way, they can manage their joint health while taking care of themselves and their growing baby.

# Exploring the basics of osteoarthritis: causes, symptoms, and impact

Osteoarthritis, often referred to as OA, is one of the most prevalent joint conditions that affects millions of individuals worldwide. It's a chronic condition that primarily targets the joints, gradually causing discomfort, pain, and changes in joint structure over time. While often associated with aging, osteoarthritis can affect people of all ages and backgrounds.

## Causes and Development

Osteoarthritis is influenced by a mix of factors:

- age plays a role, as

- wear and tear on joints over time can lead to cartilage deterioration.

- genetics contribute too, with a family history increasing vulnerability.

- joint injuries, repetitive strain, and misalignment can accelerate its onset.

- Metabolic conditions,

- sedentary habits, and

- excess weight also heightens the risk, impacting joint health.

Understanding the intricate blend of causes is key. Aging and genetics set the stage, while lifestyle and medical factors interact. Preventive steps, such as staying active, maintaining a healthy weight, and seeking early treatment for joint injuries, can help mitigate risks. Through this awareness, individuals can proactively manage and potentially delay the impact of osteoarthritis on their joint health.

## Symptoms

The hallmark symptoms of osteoarthritis include:

- joint pain,
- stiffness
- reduced flexibility
- joint tenderness
- joint swelling
- crunching or grinding sensation (crepitus) when moving the affected joint
- muscle weakness
- bony enlargement
- pain aggravation with activity
- pain relief with rest

The pain might be more noticeable after periods of inactivity or during specific movements. While osteoarthritis can affect any joint, it most commonly impacts the knees, hips, hands, and spine.

## Impact on Daily Life

In addition to causing physical discomfort, osteoarthritis can significantly affect a person's daily life. Due to pain and decreased joint motion, formerly simple tasks may become difficult. Walking, climbing stairs, and even gripping objects may become difficult as a result. Therefore, the illness may have an impact on independence, emotional health, and general quality of life.

## How pregnancy can affect osteoarthritis symptoms and progression

Pregnancy introduces a unique set of changes to the body, and these changes can influence the symptoms and progression of osteoarthritis in various ways:

### 1. Hormonal Shifts

Hormonal changes during pregnancy, particularly an increase in estrogen levels, can lead to temporary improvements in osteoarthritis symptoms for some individuals. Estrogen has anti-inflammatory properties that might alleviate joint pain. However, these effects can vary, and not all pregnant individuals with osteoarthritis experience symptom relief due to hormonal shifts.

## 2.  Weight Gain

Pregnancy typically involves weight gain as the body supports the growth of the baby. This extra weight places additional stress on joints, especially weight-bearing joints like the knees and hips. For individuals with osteoarthritis, this increased load might exacerbate joint discomfort and potentially accelerate the progression of the condition.

## 3.  Joint Laxity

Pregnancy hormones can lead to increased joint laxity, making joints more flexible. While this might be beneficial for some, it can also lead to instability in joints affected by osteoarthritis. Joint laxity could potentially contribute to injury or discomfort in those areas.

## 4.  Posture Changes

As the body accommodates the growing fetus, changes in posture are common. These changes can impact the alignment of joints, potentially affecting joints that are already compromised by osteoarthritis.

## 5.  Adaptation of Activities

Pregnant individuals often adapt their physical activities to accommodate their changing bodies. While some may reduce high-impact activities that could strain joints, others might engage in gentler exercises. These adaptations can influence how osteoarthritis symptoms are experienced.

## 6. Emotional and Psychological Factors

Pregnancy can bring about emotional and psychological changes, which might influence pain perception and coping strategies. Stress and emotional well-being can impact how osteoarthritis symptoms are managed during pregnancy.

It's important to recognize that the effects of pregnancy on osteoarthritis symptoms can vary widely from person to person. Consulting with healthcare professionals who specialize in both pregnancy and joint health can provide personalized guidance on managing symptoms, staying active, and making informed choices to ensure the well-being of both the expectant mother and the developing baby.

## The importance of personalized care and multidisciplinary approaches

The importance of personalized care and multidisciplinary approaches refers to the recognition that managing a complex condition like osteoarthritis during pregnancy requires tailored strategies that take into account an individual's unique circumstances and involve collaboration among various healthcare professionals.

## Personalized Care

Every person's experience with osteoarthritis and pregnancy is different. Personalized care means that healthcare providers take the time to understand the specific challenges, symptoms, and needs of each pregnant individual with osteoarthritis. This approach ensures that the treatment and management plans are designed to suit their individual conditions. For instance, the level of pain tolerance, joint mobility, and overall health status might vary from person to person. By customizing care, healthcare providers can offer guidance that aligns with the individual's comfort and well-being.

**Multidisciplinary Approaches**

Osteoarthritis during pregnancy requires expertise from multiple healthcare disciplines. A multidisciplinary approach involves a team of professionals with different specialties working together to provide comprehensive care. This can include obstetricians, rheumatologists (specializing in joint conditions), orthopedic specialists, physical therapists, nutritionists, and even mental health professionals.

These experts collaborate to address various aspects of health – from managing joint pain and adapting exercise routines to making safe medication choices and addressing emotional well-being. By combining their insights and skills, the team ensures a holistic and effective approach to managing both osteoarthritis and pregnancy.

Certainly, here are the key points highlighting the importance of personalized care and multidisciplinary approaches for managing osteoarthritis during pregnancy:

1. **Tailored Treatment:** Each individual's experience with osteoarthritis and pregnancy is unique. Personalized care ensures that treatment plans are specifically designed to

address the individual's symptoms, challenges, and preferences, optimizing the effectiveness of interventions.

2. **Optimal Pain Management:** Osteoarthritis can cause varying degrees of pain, and pain management strategies need to be customized. Personalized care allows healthcare providers to recommend pain relief options that align with the individual's comfort level and medical history.

3. **Risk Mitigation:** Pregnancy introduces new factors that may influence osteoarthritis symptoms. A personalized approach considers the potential impact of hormonal changes, weight gain, and joint laxity, helping to mitigate risks and enhance joint health.

4. **Safety and Efficacy:** With multiple healthcare professionals collaborating, treatment plans can be carefully coordinated to ensure safety for both the pregnant individual and the developing baby. Expert insights contribute to making informed decisions regarding medications, exercises, and interventions.

5. **Holistic Well-Being:** Osteoarthritis and pregnancy affect physical, emotional, and mental well-being. A multidisciplinary team addresses these diverse aspects of health, offering comprehensive support for managing joint pain, emotional challenges, and overall quality of life.

6. **Comprehensive Expertise:** Each healthcare professional brings specialized knowledge to the table. Obstetricians understand pregnancy, rheumatologists are experts in joint conditions, physical therapists offer tailored exercises, and

nutritionists provide dietary guidance. Combining these skills optimizes care.

7. **Adaptability:** Pregnancy is a dynamic journey, and symptoms can change over time. A personalized approach allows for adjustments in treatment strategies based on the individual's evolving needs, ensuring continuous care.

8. **Empowerment:** Personalized care empowers pregnant individuals with osteoarthritis to actively participate in their health management. It involves shared decision-making, where individuals collaborate with healthcare providers to make choices that align with their values and goals.

9. **Enhanced Quality of Life:** By addressing physical discomfort, emotional challenges, and joint health, personalized care and multidisciplinary approaches contribute to an improved overall quality of life during pregnancy.

10. **Long-Term Benefits:** The strategies and insights gained from personalized care and collaboration with a multidisciplinary team can have lasting benefits beyond pregnancy, supporting joint health and well-being throughout a person's life.

In summary, personalized care and multidisciplinary approaches prioritize individual needs, harness collective expertise, and offer a comprehensive approach to managing osteoarthritis during pregnancy. This approach not only improves symptom management but also enhances the overall pregnancy experience and lays the foundation for lifelong joint health.

# Chapter 2

## Preparing for Pregnancy with Osteoarthritis

Preparing for pregnancy with osteoarthritis involves careful planning and coordination with your healthcare team. It's important to discuss your condition and any medications you're taking with your doctors, including an obstetrician and a rheumatologist. They can help you manage pain, adjust medications if needed, and monitor your health during pregnancy. Maintaining a healthy lifestyle through proper nutrition, exercise, and managing stress can also contribute to a smoother pregnancy experience. Always follow your healthcare provider's guidance to ensure the best outcomes for both you and your baby.

### Consultation with healthcare professionals: OB-GYN, rheumatologist, and orthopedic specialist

Working with a group of medical experts, such as an orthopedic surgeon, rheumatologist, and OB-GYN, can give you comprehensive treatment and support during your pregnancy while managing your osteoarthritis.

## 1.  OB-GYN (Obstetrician-Gynecologist)

Your OB-GYN will be your primary point of contact for prenatal care. They will monitor your overall health and the health of your developing baby. They can offer guidance on nutrition, prenatal vitamins, exercise, and any specific precautions you might need to take due to your osteoarthritis. Regular check-ups will help ensure that both you and your baby are progressing well.

## 2.  Rheumatologist

Treatment of musculoskeletal diseases, such as osteoarthritis, is a specialty of your rheumatologist. To make sure your pregnancy is safe, they will evaluate your existing drug schedule and make any required adjustments. To reduce any possible dangers to the unborn child, some treatments for osteoarthritis that are often used may need to be changed during pregnancy. In order to balance pregnancy safety and pain management, your rheumatologist can work closely with your OB-GYN.

## 3.  Orthopedic Specialist

When treating osteoarthritis during pregnancy, an orthopedic specialist will concentrate on the physical side of things. They can give you tips on how to reduce joint pain, increase mobility, and make sure your joints are properly supported. They might suggest physical activity, physical therapy, or assistive technology to help you maintain your standard of living while you're expecting.

It's critical to be open and honest with every member of your healthcare team about any worries, symptoms, or changes you may be having. They can work together to develop a unique strategy that takes into account your unique demands and circumstances. This collaborative approach will not only help you manage your osteoarthritis efficiently, but it will also make sure that you and your unborn child have a better and safer pregnancy. Remember that a good pregnancy journey will involve attending appointments on time, following medical recommendations, and putting an emphasis on self-care.

## Medication management and safety considerations

It's important to carefully assess the osteoarthritis drugs you take throughout pregnancy to make sure both you and your unborn child are safe from harm. This is part of medication management and safety considerations during pregnancy. This procedure entails talking with your medical team about your current prescriptions, weighing the benefits and dangers, and modifying your drug schedule as appropriate.

The objective is to properly manage your osteoarthritis symptoms while limiting any potential risk to the unborn child. Your healthcare professionals will assist you in making knowledgeable decisions regarding the use of medications and, if necessary, may offer alternate pain management techniques. Throughout your pregnancy, regular checkups and communication with your medical team are crucial.

Here are some key points to consider:

1.  **Consultation:** Always consult your healthcare team before making any changes to your medication regimen. This includes your rheumatologist, OB-GYN, and any other relevant specialists.

2.  **Medication Review:** Your rheumatologist will review your current medications to identify which ones are safe during pregnancy. Some medications might need to be adjusted or substituted to minimize risks to the developing baby.

3.  **Risk-Benefit Analysis:** Your healthcare providers will weigh the potential benefits of medication against any potential risks to the pregnancy. Some medications may be necessary to manage your osteoarthritis symptoms, but adjustments might be needed to ensure the baby's well-being.

4.  **Pain Management:** Non-pharmacological pain management techniques, such as physical therapy, exercises, and heat/cold therapy, might be recommended to reduce reliance on medications.

5.  **Safe Medications:** Some medications, like acetaminophen, are generally considered safe during pregnancy for pain relief. However, it's crucial to use even these medications under medical guidance.

6.  **NSAIDs and Corticosteroids:** Nonsteroidal anti-inflammatory drugs (NSAIDs) and corticosteroids, commonly used for osteoarthritis, might have potential

risks during pregnancy. Your healthcare provider will advise on their safe use or alternatives.

7. **Folic Acid and Supplements:** If certain medications interfere with nutrient absorption, your healthcare provider might recommend additional supplements, such as folic acid.

8. **Timing and Dosage:** The timing and dosage of medications might need adjustment to minimize potential impact on the baby's development.

9. **Breastfeeding Considerations:** If you plan to breastfeed, discuss medication safety with your healthcare team, as some medications can pass into breast milk.

10. **Regular Monitoring:** Regular check-ups with your healthcare providers will help monitor your health and the baby's development, ensuring that any changes in your condition are addressed promptly.

Remember, the safety of both you and your baby is the top priority. Open communication with your healthcare team and strict adherence to their guidance will help ensure a healthy pregnancy while managing osteoarthritis.

**Lifestyle adjustments to support a healthy pregnancy journey**

"Lifestyle adjustments to support a healthy pregnancy journey" refers to making modifications to your regular routines and behaviors in order to provide a secure and satisfying pregnancy while also taking osteoarthritis into consideration. These modifications, which cover things like nutrition, exercise, rest, stress management, and contact with your healthcare practitioner, are meant to improve both your general wellbeing and the wellbeing of your unborn child.

Here are some key points:

### 1.  Nutrition

Focus on a well-balanced diet rich in nutrients. Include a variety of fruits, vegetables, whole grains, lean proteins, and dairy products. Consult a nutritionist for personalized advice, especially if you're on a special diet due to your osteoarthritis.

### 2.  Exercise

Engage in gentle exercises approved by your healthcare team. Activities like walking, swimming, and prenatal yoga can help maintain joint flexibility and overall fitness. Consult your healthcare provider before starting any new exercise routine.

### 3.  Weight Management

Maintain a healthy weight to reduce stress on your joints. Work with your healthcare team to determine a suitable weight gain goal during pregnancy.

### 4.  Rest and Sleep

Ensure you're getting enough rest and quality sleep. Proper sleep supports your body's healing and recovery processes.

### 5.  Hydration

Stay adequately hydrated to support your body's functions and joint health.

### 6. Stress Management

Practice relaxation techniques such as deep breathing, meditation, or prenatal massages to manage stress, which can impact both your well-being and the pregnancy.

### 7. Joint Support

Use assistive devices, such as braces or supports, as recommended by your orthopedic specialist, to ease joint discomfort.

### 8. Avoid Overexertion

Listen to your body and avoid activities that strain your joints. Ask for help when needed.

### 9. Medication Management

Follow your healthcare provider's guidance on medications. Some medications might need adjustments during pregnancy.

### 10. Regular Check-ups

Attend prenatal appointments as scheduled to monitor your health and the baby's development.

### 11. Communication

Keep an open line of communication with your healthcare team, sharing any changes in your condition or concerns.

### 12. Educate Yourself

Learn about pregnancy and osteoarthritis to make informed decisions. Attend prenatal classes and read reliable resources.

Remember, every pregnancy is unique. Your healthcare team will guide you based on your individual circumstances. By making these lifestyle adjustments, you can create a supportive environment for a healthier pregnancy while managing osteoarthritis.

# Chapter 3

## Nutritional Guidance for Joint Health

"Nutritional guidance for joint health" simply means recommendations and advice regarding the types of foods and nutrients that can help maintain and improve the health of your joints. When following nutritional guidance for joint health, you would focus on incorporating foods that are known to have anti-inflammatory properties, provide essential vitamins and minerals, and support the overall well-being of your joints.

This guidance can play a significant role in managing conditions like osteoarthritis, as certain nutrients may help reduce inflammation, support cartilage health, and alleviate joint discomfort. Consulting with a healthcare professional or nutritionist can provide you with personalized recommendations tailored to your specific needs and health goals.

### The role of a balanced diet in managing osteoarthritis during pregnancy

A balanced diet is one that includes sufficient levels of all the nutrients needed for healthy development as well as for effective everyday activities and functions. A balanced diet includes the right ratios and amounts of the nutrients required to maintain optimum health. Carbohydrates, lipids, proteins, vitamins, minerals, and water intake all need to be consumed in the right ratios and proportions.

A balanced diet plays a crucial role in managing osteoarthritis during pregnancy by providing essential nutrients that support joint health and overall well-being.

The role includes:

### 1. Inflammation Reduction

A diet rich in anti-inflammatory foods, such as fruits, vegetables, whole grains, fatty fish (rich in omega-3 fatty acids), and nuts, can help reduce inflammation associated with osteoarthritis. This can lead to decreased joint pain and discomfort.

### 2. Cartilage Support

Certain nutrients, like vitamin C, vitamin D, and antioxidants, play a role in maintaining and repairing cartilage, which is crucial for joint health. Incorporating foods high in these nutrients can aid in preserving joint function.

### 3. Weight Management

A balanced diet helps you manage your weight effectively. Maintaining a healthy weight is important for reducing stress on your joints, which is especially significant during pregnancy and when dealing with osteoarthritis.

### 4. Bone Health

Adequate intake of calcium and vitamin D is essential for strong bones. Osteoarthritis can sometimes affect bone health, so ensuring you're getting these nutrients helps support both your joints and bones.

### 5. Vital Nutrients

Protein, iron, and other essential vitamins and minerals are important for your overall health during pregnancy. Including lean protein sources, iron-rich foods, and a variety of nutrient-rich foods ensures your body gets what it needs.

### 6. Energy Levels

Pregnancy can be physically demanding, and a balanced diet provides the energy needed to cope with the changes in your body.

### 7. Digestive Health

A diet high in fiber from fruits, vegetables, and whole grains supports digestive health, preventing issues that might exacerbate discomfort from osteoarthritis.

### 8. Hydration

Staying hydrated supports joint lubrication and overall bodily functions.

Remember, each person's dietary needs are unique. It's important to work with your healthcare team or a registered dietitian to create a personalized nutrition plan that considers both your pregnancy requirements and osteoarthritis management. They can guide you in making food choices that optimize your joint health and contribute to a healthier pregnancy journey.

## Foods rich in nutrients that promote joint health

Here are some foods that are rich in nutrients known to promote joint health:

1. **Fatty Fish:** Salmon, mackerel, and sardines are high in omega-3 fatty acids, which have anti-inflammatory properties and can help reduce joint pain and stiffness.

2. **Berries:** Blueberries, strawberries, and cherries contain antioxidants that can help reduce inflammation and oxidative stress in the body.

3. **Leafy Greens:** Spinach, kale, and Swiss chard are rich in vitamins like vitamin C, which supports collagen production for healthy joints.

4. **Nuts and Seeds:** Walnuts, flaxseeds, and chia seeds provide omega-3 fatty acids, antioxidants, and fiber that support joint health.

5. **Citrus Fruits:** Oranges, lemons, and grapefruits are high in vitamin C, which plays a role in collagen synthesis and cartilage health.

6. **Turmeric:** This spice contains curcumin, a compound with potent anti-inflammatory effects that can help alleviate joint pain.

7. **Ginger:** Ginger has anti-inflammatory properties that can help reduce pain and swelling in the joints.

8. **Green Tea:** Green tea contains antioxidants that may have anti-inflammatory effects, contributing to joint health.

9. **Broccoli:** Rich in vitamins K and C, as well as sulforaphane, which has been shown to have anti-inflammatory and antioxidant effects.

10. **Beans and Legumes:** Lentils, chickpeas, and black beans are good sources of protein and fiber, which contribute to overall health and weight management.

11. **Dairy or Fortified Plant-Based Milk:** Dairy products and fortified plant-based milk provide calcium and vitamin D, essential for bone health.

12. **Lean Proteins:** Chicken, turkey, and lean cuts of red meat provide protein for muscle health, which supports joint stability.

Remember, a balanced diet that includes a variety of these nutrient-rich foods is key. Consult with a healthcare professional or a registered dietitian to create a personalized dietary plan that suits your individual needs, especially during pregnancy and while managing osteoarthritis.

## Safe and effective supplementation for expecting mothers with osteoarthritis

Obstetricians, gynecologists, rheumatologists, and certified dietitians should all be consulted before supplementation for pregnant women with osteoarthritis is started.

Here are some considerations for safe and effective supplementation:

1. **Folic Acid**

Folic acid is crucial for fetal development. Your healthcare provider might recommend prenatal vitamins containing folic acid to reduce the risk of certain birth defects.

2. **Vitamin D**

Adequate vitamin D is essential for bone health. If you have limited sun exposure or are at risk of deficiency, your healthcare provider might recommend vitamin D supplements.

3. **Calcium**

Calcium supports both your bone health and the developing baby's skeletal growth. Your healthcare team can guide you on the appropriate intake and potential need for supplementation.

4. **Omega-3 Fatty Acids**

Omega-3s from fish oil supplements might help reduce inflammation and support joint health. Consult your healthcare provider for guidance on suitable dosages.

5. **Iron**

Iron is important for preventing anemia during pregnancy. Your healthcare provider will monitor your iron levels and recommend supplements if needed.

6. **Vitamin B12**

If you follow a vegetarian or vegan diet, you might need vitamin B12 supplementation, as this vitamin is primarily found in animal products.

### 7. Avoid Over-Supplementation

Taking excessive amounts of certain vitamins and minerals can be harmful. Stick to the recommended dosages and seek guidance.

### 8. Balanced Diet First

Supplements should complement a healthy diet, not replace it. Focus on obtaining nutrients from whole foods whenever possible.

### 9. Quality and Safety

Choose supplements from reputable brands that undergo third-party testing for quality and safety.

### 10. Consultation

Always consult your healthcare team before starting any supplements. They will consider your individual health, dietary habits, and potential interactions with other medications.

Remember that every pregnancy is unique, and your healthcare team will tailor recommendations to your specific needs. Don't start or stop any supplements without consulting your healthcare provider, as they will ensure that your supplementation plan aligns with both your pregnancy and osteoarthritis management goals.

# Chapter 4

## Physical Activity and Exercises

Physical activity and exercises, refer to staying active through various movements and workouts. This is important for maintaining good health, managing conditions like osteoarthritis, and supporting a healthy pregnancy.

It's important to speak with your healthcare providers before beginning any fitness program if you are pregnant and have osteoarthritis. Focus on exercises that can keep your joints and body in good form, such as walking, swimming, and light weight training. Always pay attention to your body, steer clear of demanding tasks, and put your comfort and security first. Better joint health and general wellbeing can be attributed to staying active throughout pregnancy.

**Tailored exercise routines to alleviate joint pain and stiffness**

Tailored exercise routines are customized workout plans designed specifically for an individual's unique needs, goals, and circumstances. These routines are created based on factors such as your health condition, fitness level, any existing medical conditions (like osteoarthritis), pregnancy status, and personal preferences.

Tailored exercise routines can be beneficial for alleviating joint pain and stiffness, especially for individuals dealing with conditions like osteoarthritis.

Here's how they work:

### 1. Individualized Approach

A tailored exercise routine is designed specifically for you, taking into account your health status, joint condition, pregnancy, and any other considerations.

### 2. Low-Impact Exercises

These routines often include low-impact exercises that are gentle on your joints, such as walking, swimming, and cycling. These activities help improve circulation, reduce stiffness, and maintain joint flexibility.

### 3. Range of Motion Exercises

Gentle stretches and range of motion exercises can improve joint mobility and flexibility. These movements help counteract stiffness and discomfort. Examples are:

- neck rotations, shoulder circles, arm swings,

- wrist flexibility exercises, ankle circles, hip rotations,

- knee extensions, toe flexibility movements, spine flexion and extension, and

- pelvic tilts.

## 4. Strengthening Exercises

Targeted strength training can help stabilize joints and support the muscles surrounding them. Strengthening exercises can reduce strain on your joints and improve overall joint function.

Examples include:

- pelvic floor contractions (Kegel exercises) to support the pelvic region,

- squats for lower body strength,

- leg lifts for targeted leg muscles,

- arm raises and bicep curls to work the upper body,

- wall push-ups for arm and chest strength,

- modified planks to engage core muscles,

- seated rows for back and arm muscles,

- step-ups for leg strength, and

- pelvic tilts to engage the abdominal region.

## 5. Core Exercises

Strengthening your core muscles can provide better support to your spine and improve posture, which can alleviate pressure on your joints.

Examples:

- pelvic tilts, modified planks,

- seated leg lifts, bridge lifts, cat-cow stretch,

- side leg raises, standing torso twist,

- sitting rotations, dead bug and coobra stretch.

### 6. Balancing Exercises

Balance-focused exercises help enhance stability, reducing the risk of falls and supporting joint alignment.

### 7. Progressive Approach

Tailored routines often start with manageable exercises and gradually progress as your body adapts and becomes stronger.

### 8. Pregnancy Considerations

When pregnant, exercises are modified to accommodate your changing body. Some poses or movements might need to be avoided to ensure the safety of both you and your baby.

### 9. Supervised Training

If possible, consider working with a fitness professional experienced in working with pregnant individuals and those with osteoarthritis. They can provide guidance and ensure that exercises are performed correctly.

### 10. Consistency

Regular practice of your tailored routine is key. Consistency helps maintain joint flexibility and muscle strength, leading to long-term benefits.

Remember that each person's needs are unique. Always consult your healthcare providers before starting any new exercise routine, especially during pregnancy and when managing a condition like osteoarthritis. A personalized approach will ensure that you're engaging in exercises that are safe, effective, and well-suited to your situation.

# Low-impact activities suitable for pregnant individuals with osteoarthritis

Certainly, low-impact activities are generally suitable and safe for pregnant individuals with osteoarthritis, as they minimize stress on the joints while providing cardiovascular and overall health benefits.

Here are some low-impact activities you might consider:

1. **Walking:** Walking is a gentle and accessible exercise that can be done at your own pace. It helps improve cardiovascular health, maintain joint flexibility, and boost your mood.

2. **Swimming:** Swimming and water aerobics are excellent options for pregnant individuals with osteoarthritis. The buoyancy of the water reduces impact on joints while providing a full-body workout.

3. **Cycling:** Stationary cycling or using a recumbent bike is a low-impact way to improve cardiovascular fitness without putting excess strain on your joints.

4. **Prenatal Yoga:** Prenatal yoga classes are tailored to the needs of pregnant individuals. Yoga helps improve flexibility, balance, and relaxation, which can be particularly beneficial during pregnancy and while managing osteoarthritis.

5. **Tai Chi:** Tai Chi is a gentle form of exercise that focuses on slow, flowing movements. It helps improve balance, coordination, and relaxation.

6. **Elliptical Trainer:** Using an elliptical machine provides a low-impact cardio workout, promoting joint health while engaging both upper and lower body muscles.

7. **Low-impact Aerobics:** Some aerobic classes are specifically designed for pregnant individuals and those with joint conditions. These classes incorporate gentle movements to improve cardiovascular fitness.

8. **Strength Training with Resistance Bands:** Using resistance bands can provide a low-impact way to strengthen muscles without putting excessive stress on your joints.

9. **Stretching:** Incorporate gentle stretching exercises to maintain flexibility and alleviate joint stiffness.

Always consult your healthcare provider before starting any new exercise routine, especially during pregnancy and when managing osteoarthritis. They can guide you on the most suitable activities based on your individual health needs and help ensure a safe and comfortable workout experience.

## Expert guidance on maintaining fitness while safeguarding your joints and pregnancy

Expert advice on being fit while protecting your joints and becoming pregnant requires a multifaceted strategy that combines the knowledge of healthcare professionals and fitness experts. To have a firm understanding of your pregnancy and osteoarthritis situation, speak with your OB-GYN, rheumatologist, and orthopedic doctor first. Their advice will pave the path for a personalized exercise program that takes into account your particular requirements and difficulties.

Work with a trained fitness professional with knowledge of joint health during pregnancy to develop a training schedule that achieves the proper balance between remaining active and safeguarding your joints. This strategy makes sure that every workout you do is carefully selected to reduce joint stress and enhance overall fitness.

Include low-impact exercises like walking, swimming, and prenatal yoga since they improve your heart health without putting undue strain on your joints. During workouts, concentrate on maintaining perfect form to avoid needless strain and lower the risk of injury.

Frequent check-ins with your medical team allow for ongoing evaluation of your health and the need for any necessary alterations to your workout routine. Staying hydrated, eating a balanced diet, and managing discomfort with efficient pain management approaches are essential to supporting both your joint health and your pregnancy.

Following expert advice eventually gives you the ability to create an exercise routine that protects and prioritizes both your health and the health of your unborn child.

# Chapter 5

# Pain Management and Coping Strategies

"Pain management and coping strategies" refers to the approaches and strategies people take to address and lessen physical pain as well as deal with the potential emotional and psychological effects that pain may have. This idea entails figuring out how to control joint pain and discomfort while managing the particular difficulties of pregnancy for women with osteoarthritis.

## Pain Management

These are approaches aimed at reducing or controlling physical pain. This could involve taking prescribed medications that are safe during pregnancy, using heat or cold therapy, doing specific exercises or stretches to improve joint function, and utilizing assistive devices like braces or splints to support the affected joints.

## Coping Strategies

Coping strategies are ways to handle the emotional and mental aspects of pain. They help individuals manage the stress, anxiety, and frustration that can come with experiencing pain. This might include mindfulness practices to stay present and manage pain-related stress, seeking support from friends, family, or support groups, engaging in activities that distract from the pain, and using positive thinking to maintain a hopeful outlook despite the discomfort.

These techniques are particularly crucial when it comes to pregnancy and osteoarthritis since they not only assist people deal with physical discomfort but also keep their emotional wellbeing while going through a time of great change and difficulty. It's essential to collaborate with healthcare professionals to create a specialized plan that includes these techniques in a method that is secure and efficient for managing osteoarthritis symptoms as well as pregnancy.

### Non-pharmacological pain relief methods: heat therapy, acupuncture, and more

Non-pharmacological pain relief methods refer to techniques and approaches that don't involve medication to manage pain.

Here are some examples:

1. **Heat Therapy:** Applying heat to sore joints can help relax muscles, improve blood flow, and provide relief. You can use warm towels, heating pads, or warm baths for localized comfort.

2. **Cold Therapy:** Cold packs or ice wrapped in a cloth can reduce inflammation and numb the area, temporarily easing pain and swelling.

3. **Acupuncture:** This traditional Chinese therapy involves inserting thin needles into specific points on the body. Some people find it helpful for managing pain, including joint discomfort.

4. **Massage Therapy:** Gentle massage can reduce muscle tension and promote relaxation. However, ensure the therapist is experienced with prenatal massage if you're pregnant.

5. **Physical Therapy:** A physical therapist can design exercises and stretches tailored to your needs, helping improve joint mobility and strength while managing pain.

6. **Yoga and Stretching:** Gentle yoga poses and stretches can help increase flexibility, improve posture, and alleviate muscle tension associated with joint pain.

7. **Mindfulness and Meditation:** Techniques such as deep breathing, mindfulness, and meditation can help manage pain perception and reduce stress.

8. **Hydrotherapy:** Immersing yourself in a warm pool can relieve pressure on joints and promote relaxation. This is particularly beneficial during pregnancy.

9. **TENS (Transcutaneous Electrical Nerve Stimulation):** This involves using a small device to deliver mild electrical currents to the skin, which can help reduce pain signals.

10. **Supportive Devices:** Orthotic devices like braces, splints, or crutches can provide support to joints, reducing strain and discomfort.

11. **Biofeedback:** This technique teaches you to control certain body functions, such as muscle tension, through relaxation techniques.

12. **Cognitive Behavioral Therapy (CBT):** CBT helps manage pain by addressing negative thought patterns and promoting coping strategies.

Remember, it's important to consult your healthcare providers before trying any new pain relief methods, especially during pregnancy and when dealing with osteoarthritis. They can guide you on which approaches are safe and suitable for your individual situation.

## Mindfulness and relaxation techniques to reduce stress and improve well-being

Mindfulness and relaxation techniques are practices that can help reduce stress, enhance well-being, and promote a sense of calm and balance.

Here's how they work:

### Mindfulness Techniques

Mindfulness involves being fully present and aware of the present moment without judgment. It can help you manage stress and improve your overall mental and emotional state.

Techniques include:

1.  **Deep Breathing:** Focusing on your breath can help bring your attention to the present moment and calm your mind.

2.  **Body Scan:** Mentally scan your body, paying attention to any sensations or tension. This helps you become aware of how your body feels and promotes relaxation.

3.  **Mindful Eating:** Eating slowly and savoring each bite can enhance your enjoyment of food and help you connect with your senses.

4.  **Mindful Walking:** While walking, pay attention to each step, your surroundings, and the sensations in your body.

5.  **Meditation:** Meditation involves focusing your attention on a specific object, thought, or breath, helping you cultivate a sense of calm and clarity.

## Relaxation Techniques

Relaxation techniques aim to reduce physical and mental tension. These practices can help manage pain, improve sleep, and enhance overall well-being.

Examples include:

1.  **Progressive Muscle Relaxation:** This involves tensing and then relaxing different muscle groups in your body to release tension.

2. **Guided Imagery:** Visualization of peaceful or calming scenes can help reduce stress and induce relaxation.

3. **Autogenic Training:** Using self-suggestion, you repeat certain phrases to promote relaxation and well-being.

4. **Breathing Exercises: Controlled** breathing techniques can help slow your heart rate and ease tension.

5. **Yoga and Tai Chi:** These practices combine movement, breath, and meditation to promote relaxation and flexibility.

By incorporating mindfulness and relaxation techniques into your daily routine, you can effectively manage stress, promote a positive mindset, and improve your overall quality of life. Whether you're pregnant or dealing with osteoarthritis, these practices can offer valuable support to your well-being. If you're new to these techniques, consider exploring classes, apps, or online resources to learn and practice them effectively.

**Building a strong support network for emotional and physical support**

Building a strong support network involves creating a circle of individuals who provide both emotional and physical support during challenging times such as pregnancy while managing osteoarthritis.

Here's how it works:

## Emotional Support

1. **Family and Friends:** Reach out to loved ones who can lend a listening ear, offer encouragement, and share your journey.

2. **Support Groups:** Join online or in-person support groups for pregnant individuals with osteoarthritis. Connecting with others who understand your situation can be comforting.

3. **Therapists or Counselors:** Professional therapists can provide a safe space to discuss your feelings and develop coping strategies.

4. **Healthcare Providers:** Your OB-GYN, rheumatologist, and orthopedic specialist can offer medical guidance as well as emotional support during your pregnancy.

5. **Pregnancy Classes:** Attending prenatal classes provides an opportunity to connect with other expectant parents and share experiences.

## Physical Support

1. **Partner or Spouse:** Your partner can provide physical help with daily tasks, offer massages, and be a source of comfort.

2. **Family Members:** Relatives can assist with household chores, groceries, and caring for older children.

3.  **Friends:** Close friends can lend a hand with tasks, offer rides to appointments, and provide practical assistance.

4.  **Healthcare Providers:** Your medical team can offer guidance on managing physical challenges while pregnant with osteoarthritis.

5.  **Fitness Professionals:** Certified trainers can help design safe exercise routines that align with your pregnancy and joint health needs.

Having a strong support network can alleviate stress, reduce feelings of isolation, and enhance your overall well-being. Communicate openly with your support system about your needs and how they can best help you. Remember, seeking support is a sign of strength, and creating a network of understanding individuals can positively impact your pregnancy journey while managing osteoarthritis.

# Chapter 6

## Navigating Pregnancy Milestones with Osteoarthritis

The phrase "navigating pregnancy milestones with osteoarthritis" refers to the act of managing the various phases and events of pregnancy with the difficulties osteoarthritis presents. To achieve a healthy and enjoyable pregnancy, it requires careful planning, talking with medical professionals, and making adjustments to your habits and tactics.

This strategy includes dealing with joint pain, modifying exercise routines, talking about pain control during labor, and figuring out how to take care of both you and your child while taking osteoarthritis into account. People with osteoarthritis can still have a good and well-managed pregnancy journey by carefully navigating these milestones and with professional assistance.

They are as follows:

**Prenatal Care and Planning**

1. **Consult Healthcare Providers:** Early on, consult your OB-GYN, rheumatologist, and orthopedic specialist to create a comprehensive plan that addresses both your pregnancy and osteoarthritis needs.

2. **Medication Review:** Review your medications with your healthcare team. They will determine which ones are safe during pregnancy and make any necessary adjustments.

## First Trimester

1. **Fatigue and Pain Management:** Fatigue is common in the first trimester. Prioritize rest, and continue using pain management strategies that are safe for pregnancy.

2. **Nutrition and Hydration:** Focus on a balanced diet and stay hydrated. Consult a nutritionist if needed.

## Second Trimester

1. **Exercise:** Engage in safe exercises approved by your healthcare provider. Low-impact activities and tailored routines can help manage joint pain.

2. **Body Changes:** As your body changes, adjust your exercise routines, and consider using supportive devices if needed.

## Third Trimester

1. **Preparation:** Plan for labor and postpartum needs. Discuss pain management strategies during delivery with your healthcare team.

2. **Joint Support:** Use pillows and supports to ease joint discomfort during sleep. Maintain gentle exercise to improve flexibility and strength.

## Labor and Delivery

1. Pain **Management:** Work with your medical team to create a pain management plan that considers your osteoarthritis and ensures a comfortable labor experience.

2. **Mobility Aids:** If needed, have mobility aids available during labor to help with movement and positioning.

## Postpartum Period

1. **Recovery:** Allow yourself time to recover after delivery. Gradually reintroduce exercises after receiving approval from your healthcare provider.

2. **Self-Care:** Prioritize self-care to manage joint pain and support your well-being as a new parent.

## Baby Care

1. **Body Mechanics:** Use ergonomic techniques when lifting and carrying your baby to minimize strain on your joints.

Ergonomic techniques involve adjusting your body posture and the way you interact with objects and your environment to minimize physical strain and discomfort.

In the context of pregnancy and managing osteoarthritis, ergonomic techniques can be especially useful to reduce joint pain and support your overall well-being. These techniques aim to create a comfortable and efficient environment that promotes healthy body mechanics and reduces the risk of injury or discomfort.

Examples include maintaining proper posture while sitting, using supportive cushions, adjusting the height of work surfaces to reduce strain, and using tools and equipment that promote ease of movement and minimize joint stress.

2.  **Support Network:** Lean on your support network for assistance with baby care tasks.

Remember, communication with your healthcare team and support network is key. Be adaptable and listen to your body's cues. By collaborating with professionals and incorporating strategies that prioritize both your pregnancy and osteoarthritis management, you can navigate these milestones with confidence and care.

## First trimester challenges: morning sickness, fatigue, and joint pain

The first trimester of pregnancy often comes with a set of challenges that can impact your well-being, especially when dealing with osteoarthritis.

Here's a brief overview of these challenges:

### 1. **Morning Sickness**

Many pregnant individuals experience nausea and vomiting, commonly referred to as morning sickness. While it's not limited to the mornings, it can occur at any time of day. Managing morning sickness involves eating small, frequent meals, staying hydrated, avoiding strong odors, and finding foods that are gentle on your stomach. If you're also managing osteoarthritis, it's important to choose easily digestible foods that provide essential nutrients for joint health.

### 2. **Fatigue**

The surge in hormone levels during the first trimester can lead to increased fatigue. Your body is working hard to support the developing baby. Adequate rest and sleep are crucial during this time. Listen to your body, and don't hesitate to take naps or rest when needed. Managing fatigue while dealing with osteoarthritis may require adjusting your daily routine and making time for relaxation and gentle movement to prevent joint stiffness.

### 3. **Joint Pain**

If you're already dealing with osteoarthritis, the hormonal changes of pregnancy can impact your joints further. Hormones that loosen ligaments for childbirth can also affect joint stability. Gentle exercises, such as range of motion and low-impact activities approved by your healthcare provider, can help maintain joint mobility. Heat or cold therapy, and using assistive devices if necessary, can alleviate joint pain while considering your pregnancy.

Navigating these challenges requires a balance of self-care, proper nutrition, and consulting your healthcare providers for guidance tailored to your pregnancy and osteoarthritis needs. Remember that each pregnancy is unique, so what works best for you may vary.

## Second trimester: adapting to body changes and maintaining mobility

During the second trimester of pregnancy, adapting to body changes and maintaining mobility become key considerations, especially if you're managing osteoarthritis.

Here's a concise overview:

### 1. Body Changes

As your baby grows, your body undergoes various changes. Your abdomen expands, which can affect your center of gravity and posture. Adapt to these changes by choosing supportive clothing and footwear. Maternity belts or bands can offer additional support to your lower back and pelvis. Consider discussing body changes with your healthcare provider to ensure that your osteoarthritis management plan remains effective.

### 2. Maintaining Mobility

The second trimester is often referred to as the "honeymoon phase" of pregnancy, as many women experience increased energy levels. Capitalize on this by engaging in safe and gentle exercises approved by your healthcare provider. Low-impact activities like swimming, walking, and prenatal yoga can help maintain joint flexibility and overall mobility. Focus on proper body mechanics and alignment to reduce strain on your joints.

### 3. Stretching and Flexibility

Incorporate regular stretching routines to alleviate muscle tension and improve flexibility. Gentle stretches can help with joint mobility and reduce discomfort. Consult your healthcare provider or a certified fitness professional for guidance on safe stretching exercises that suit your pregnancy and osteoarthritis condition.

Remember that your body's response to pregnancy and osteoarthritis is unique. Consult your healthcare team regularly to adapt your strategies and ensure that you're effectively managing both your pregnancy and joint health. Staying active, practicing good posture, and maintaining joint flexibility can contribute to a more comfortable and enjoyable second trimester.

## Third trimester considerations: preparing for labor, delivery, and postpartum recovery

In the third trimester of pregnancy, preparing for labor, delivery, and postpartum recovery becomes a focal point, especially when dealing with osteoarthritis.

Here's a concise overview:

### 1. Labor and Delivery Preparation

As you approach the final weeks of pregnancy, focus on preparing for labor and delivery. Discuss pain management options with your healthcare provider, taking into consideration your osteoarthritis needs. Consider creating a birth plan that outlines your preferences and any accommodations you might require due to your condition.

## 2. Joint Support

As your body continues to change, be mindful of your joint health. Use pillows and supports to alleviate joint discomfort during sleep. Engage in gentle exercises, approved by your healthcare provider, to maintain joint mobility and flexibility. Incorporate relaxation techniques to manage any stress or anxiety related to labor and delivery.

## 3. Postpartum Recovery

Plan for your postpartum recovery by setting up a comfortable space at home and arranging for support from family and friends. If you had a cesarean section, you may need to be extra cautious with lifting and movement, considering your osteoarthritis. Gradually reintroduce exercise after receiving clearance from your healthcare provider, focusing on exercises that promote joint mobility without causing strain.

## 4. Breastfeeding and Positioning

If you plan to breastfeed, explore comfortable breastfeeding positions that minimize joint strain. Use supportive pillows and cushions to maintain good posture and ease joint discomfort while nursing.

## 5. Consult Your Healthcare Provider

Regularly communicate with your healthcare team about your osteoarthritis symptoms and how they might interact with your pregnancy, labor, and postpartum experiences. They can offer guidance on pain management, exercises, and adjustments to your routine.

The third trimester is a critical time for ensuring that your joint health and pregnancy management align seamlessly. Preparing for labor, delivery, and postpartum recovery with consideration for your osteoarthritis allows you to navigate these milestones while prioritizing your well-being and comfort.

# Chapter 7

## Postpartum Care and Beyond

The phrase "postpartum care and beyond" refers to the time after delivery and the ongoing thoughts and steps that must be taken to ensure the health of both the new mother and the infant. Recovery from childbirth, coping with the physical and psychological changes that follow giving birth, and attending to the needs of the infant are all included in this phase.

For a pregnant individual managing osteoarthritis, "Postpartum Care and Beyond" also involves continuing to manage your joint health while adapting to the demands of caring for a newborn. This may include: physical recovery, emotional well-being, baby care, balancing self-care and long- term joint health.

### Managing osteoarthritis flare-ups after childbirth

Managing osteoarthritis flare-ups after childbirth involves addressing sudden increases in joint pain and inflammation that can occur due to the physical demands of childbirth and the postpartum period.

Here's how to approach this situation:

1. **Rest and Recovery:** After childbirth, prioritize rest to allow your body to recover. Avoid overexertion and give yourself time to heal.

2. **Pain Management Techniques:** Continue using pain management techniques that are safe for postpartum and breastfeeding, such as heat or cold therapy, gentle stretches, and relaxation techniques.

3. **Medication:** If you're on medications for osteoarthritis, consult your healthcare provider before resuming or adjusting any medication postpartum. Some medications may need to be modified for breastfeeding.

4. **Gentle Movement:** Engage in gentle exercises approved by your healthcare provider. These can help maintain joint mobility and prevent stiffness.

5. **Proper Body Mechanics:** Be mindful of your body mechanics when caring for your baby. Use ergonomic techniques to avoid strain on your joints while lifting, holding, and feeding.

6. **Support Network:** Lean on your support network for assistance with baby care and household tasks, especially during flare-ups when you might need more help.

7. **Consult Healthcare Providers:** If flare-ups persist or worsen, consult your healthcare providers. They can provide guidance on managing flare-ups safely and effectively.

8.  **Balanced Diet:** Maintain a balanced diet that supports your joint health and overall recovery.

Remember that flare-ups can happen due to hormonal changes, increased physical demands, and stress. It's important to listen to your body and not push yourself too hard during this time. Seek professional advice if needed to manage your osteoarthritis symptoms while adjusting to the demands of caring for a newborn.

**Balancing newborn care with self-care: practical tips for joint health**

"Balancing newborn care with self-care: practical tips for joint health" refers to the process of effectively managing the demands of caring for a newborn while also taking steps to prioritize your own well-being, particularly in relation to your joint health, especially if you're dealing with osteoarthritis.

This concept acknowledges that while caring for your baby is a top priority, it's essential to ensure that you're also looking after yourself physically and mentally. The practical tips provided in this context aim to help you strike a balance between the responsibilities of parenting and the need to maintain your own joint health and overall health.

These tips include suggestions for managing daily activities in ways that reduce strain on your joints, incorporate gentle movement, and allow for moments of relaxation and self-care, ensuring that you can care for both your baby and yourself effectively.

Here are practical tips to prioritize both:

1. **Use Supportive Tools:** Opt for baby gear that reduces strain on your joints, like ergonomic baby carriers and nursing pillows.

2. **Create Comfortable Spaces:** Set up stations around your home with supportive cushions and pillows to maintain good posture while feeding and holding the baby.

3. **Lifting Techniques:** Practice proper lifting techniques by bending your knees and using your leg muscles rather than straining your back and joints.

4. **Utilize Rest Periods:** Nap when the baby sleeps to ensure you're getting enough rest and recovery.

5. **Gentle Movement:** Incorporate gentle stretches and movement throughout the day to maintain joint mobility. Consult your healthcare provider for safe exercises.

6. **Delegate Tasks:** Enlist the help of your partner, family, and friends for tasks like diaper changes, lifting the baby, and household chores.

7. **Time Management:** Plan your day to balance baby care with self-care. Set aside moments for relaxation, stretching, and managing your osteoarthritis symptoms.

8. **Stay Hydrated and Nourished:** Maintain a balanced diet and stay hydrated to support your joint health and energy levels.

9. **Accept Help:** Don't hesitate to accept offers of assistance from loved ones. It's okay to ask for help when needed.

10. **Prioritize Rest:** Your rest and well-being are essential. Don't neglect your own needs while caring for your baby.

11. **Communicate with Healthcare Providers:** Regularly update your healthcare team about any changes in your osteoarthritis symptoms and discuss how to manage them while caring for your baby.

12. **Mindful Breathing:** Practice deep breathing techniques to manage stress and stay grounded during demanding moments.

13. **Engage in Self-Care:** Set aside time for activities you enjoy, whether it's reading, a warm bath, or a short walk.

Remember that finding a balance takes time and adjustment. Don't put too much pressure on yourself to do everything perfectly. Prioritizing both newborn care and self-care will contribute to a more manageable and fulfilling postpartum experience.

## Long-term strategies for managing osteoarthritis as you continue your parenting journey

"Long-term strategies for managing osteoarthritis as you continue your parenting journey" talks about the proactive approaches and plans you can adopt to effectively handle the challenges of parenting while also managing the ongoing symptoms and impact of osteoarthritis.

It recognizes that parenting is a lifelong commitment and that your osteoarthritis management needs to be integrated into your parenting journey for the long haul. These strategies encompass various aspects of your life, including physical well-being, emotional health, and practical considerations, ensuring that you can provide the best care for your child while prioritizing your own joint health.

As you continue your parenting journey while managing osteoarthritis, implementing these strategies over the long term can help you navigate the complexities of parenting with osteoarthritis in a way that supports both you and your child's well-being.

Here are some effective approaches:

1. **Consistent Exercise Routine:** Maintain a regular exercise routine that includes low-impact activities, stretching, and strengthening exercises. Regular movement can help manage joint pain and maintain flexibility.

2. **Healthy Diet:** Follow a balanced diet rich in nutrients that support joint health, such as omega-3 fatty acids, antioxidants, and vitamin D. Consult a nutritionist for personalized recommendations.

3. **Weight Management:** Maintain a healthy weight to reduce strain on your joints. A healthy weight can minimize the impact of osteoarthritis and support your overall well-being.

4. **Pain Management Techniques:** Continue to use safe pain management techniques, such as heat or cold therapy, gentle exercises, and relaxation techniques.

5. **Adaptable Self-Care:** Adjust your self-care routines as your child grows. Find moments for relaxation, exercise, and pain relief even amid your parenting responsibilities.

6. **Regular Check-ups:** Schedule regular appointments with your healthcare providers to monitor your osteoarthritis and receive guidance on managing your condition.

7. **Support Network:** Lean on your support network for assistance with parenting tasks and household chores when needed.

8. **Modify Activities:** Adapt your activities to your joint health. Use assistive devices if necessary, and avoid activities that exacerbate joint pain.

9. **Stress Management:** Practice stress reduction techniques, such as mindfulness, meditation, and deep breathing, to manage the demands of parenting and osteoarthritis.

10. **Open Communication:** Keep communicating with your healthcare team about your symptoms and any changes. They can adjust your treatment plan accordingly.

11. **Time Management:** Prioritize tasks, set realistic expectations, and allocate time for self-care without feeling guilty.

12. **Embrace Flexibility:** Understand that there will be ups and downs. Be adaptable and kind to yourself as you navigate your parenting journey with osteoarthritis.

13. **Positive Mindset:** Maintain a positive outlook and focus on what you can do rather than what you can't.

Remember that parenting with osteoarthritis is a journey that requires patience and self-compassion. By implementing these long-term strategies, you can continue to care for yourself and your child while effectively managing your condition.

# Chapter 8

## Real Stories, Real Inspiration

"Real Stories, Real Inspiration" highlights the value of sharing personal experiences to inspire others who may be going through similar difficulties or circumstances and to make them more relatable. It could be used to describe the sharing of personal accounts from people who have effectively treated osteoarthritis while navigating pregnancy and parenthood in this context.

These narratives can highlight the approaches, resiliency, and optimism that actual people have shown in their journeys, providing inspiration and direction for others who are facing comparable challenges. A sense of belonging, empathy, and the knowledge that people are not alone in their situations can all be fostered by sharing these true stories. It can also provide helpful insights and a feeling of hope to people who are looking for direction and comfort while managing osteoarthritis through major life transitions like pregnancy and parenthood.

# Personal anecdotes from individuals who successfully managed osteoarthritis during pregnancy

Certainly, here are a few personal anecdotes from individuals who successfully managed osteoarthritis during pregnancy:

## Anna's Story

*"During my pregnancy, my osteoarthritis flared up, and I was worried about how I would cope. But with the support of my healthcare team, I tailored my exercise routine to include gentle stretches and prenatal yoga. Connecting with other expectant moms in a support group gave me a sense of community and reassurance. It wasn't always easy, but focusing on self-care and staying positive helped me navigate both pregnancy and osteoarthritis."*

## David's Journey

*"Being a soon-to-be dad while managing osteoarthritis seemed daunting, but I knew I had to be there for my partner. I learned to communicate openly with her about my limitations, and together we found creative ways to share parenting tasks. Using assistive devices and ergonomic techniques helped me stay involved and minimize joint strain. It's been an incredible journey of teamwork and adaptation."*

**Emily's Experience**

*"When I found out I was pregnant, I was concerned about the joint pain from my osteoarthritis affecting my mobility. My healthcare providers customized a safe exercise plan, and I incorporated nutrient-rich foods to support my joints. Even when fatigue hit, I focused on pacing myself and practicing relaxation techniques. My son is now a toddler, and I'm grateful for the strategies that helped me manage my health and be a hands-on mom."*

These personal anecdotes highlight the diverse ways individuals successfully managed osteoarthritis during pregnancy. They underscore the importance of communication, support from healthcare providers, adapting routines, and embracing self-care. Each story shows that with determination and the right strategies, it's possible to navigate the challenges of pregnancy while managing osteoarthritis effectively.

## Triumphs, challenges, and lessons learned on the road to motherhood with osteoarthritis

"Triumphs, challenges, and lessons learned on the road to motherhood with osteoarthritis" encapsulates the multifaceted journey of individuals who have experienced the intersection of managing osteoarthritis while becoming mothers.

Here's what each aspect signifies:

## Triumphs

These are the successes, achievements, and positive moments that individuals experience while balancing the demands of motherhood and managing osteoarthritis. These could include moments of overcoming physical challenges, finding effective pain management strategies, and celebrating milestones with their child.

## Challenges

These represent the obstacles, difficulties, and hurdles faced by individuals dealing with osteoarthritis while becoming mothers. Challenges could include managing joint pain while caring for a newborn, adapting to changes in routine, and finding the right balance between self-care and baby care.

## Lessons Learned

These are the learnings, wisdom, and lessons learned through raising children with osteoarthritis. Lessons can include understanding the value of self-compassion, learning how to ask for assistance, developing efficient coping mechanisms, and appreciating the strength and resilience that can come from such a journey.

This phrase encapsulates the holistic and complex journey of individuals who navigate the unique path of motherhood while managing the challenges of osteoarthritis. It reflects the triumphs that come from perseverance, the challenges that arise from managing two important roles, and the valuable lessons that shape their approach to both parenting and self-care.

## Conclusion

As you embark on the remarkable journey of pregnancy with osteoarthritis, remember that you are not alone. This book serves as your companion, offering invaluable insights, expert advice, and practical tips to guide you through this unique chapter of your life. By combining medical knowledge with a holistic approach, you can navigate the challenges, celebrate the triumphs, and embrace the joys of motherhood while effectively managing osteoarthritis.

# Reference


https://my.clevelandclinic.org/health/diseases/5599-osteoarthritis

https://timesofindia.indiatimes.com/life-
style/parenting/pregnancy/lunar-eclipse-pregnancy-
precautions-chandra-grahan-me-pregnant-lady-kya-kare-
what-should-a-pregnant-woman-do-during-lunar-eclipse-
pregnancy-lunar-eclipse-effect/articleshow/79478297.cms

https://www.biologyonline.com/dictionary/balanced-diet#

https://www.cdc.gov/arthritis/basics/osteoarthritis.htm#

https://www.medicalnewstoday.com/articles/pregnancy-arthritis#

https://www.verywellhealth.com/arthritis-and-pregnancy-
5188405